Will You
(or Someone You Love)
Get Prostate Cancer?

A SURVIVOR SHEDS SOME LIGHT

John Sias

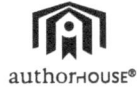

authorHOUSE®

AuthorHouse™
1663 Liberty Drive, Suite 200
Bloomington, IN 47403
www.authorhouse.com
Phone: 1-800-839-8640

The information and opinions expressed in this book are not an endorsement
or recommendation for any treatment, service or course of action. For medical
or other advice, please consult appropriate professionals of your choice. The
author is merely a survivor of prostate cancer and not a physician.

First published by AuthorHouse 11/5/2007

ISBN: 978-1-4343-4209-6 (sc)

Printed in the United States of America
Bloomington, Indiana

This book is printed on acid-free paper.

To my wife, Marie, who saved my life
the day she persuaded me
to visit the doctor

FOREWORD

On the way home after a day's skiing in January of 2001, my wife casually asked, "When was the last time you had a physical exam?" After hearing no reply and seeing a blank look on my face, she followed up with a stern demand, "Well, it's about time you had another one!"

A week after the exam, the doctor told me, "Mr. Sias, I think you should see a urologist. Your PSA is high."

I asked, "What's a urologist? And what's this thing you call PSA?" (You can see my level of medical knowledge at this time.) Probably because I'd never been seriously ill in all my life, I had little curiosity about health-related matters.

The urologist told me my PSA was 11 and a later biopsy told me I had cancer in 11 of the 12 samples he had extracted from my prostate. He said I should make a date for surgery. I was 70. This was my first PSA screening. Was surgery my only option?

Things were happening too fast. I'm not a worrier. But I knew I had a serious problem, so when I arrived home an hour later and told my wife the bad news, I said, "We need to get away and think about this situation."

After a week in the Florida Keys (a much warmer place in February to think things over than frigid New England!), we determined the first thing to do was to learn as much as we could about prostate cancer.

Having owned a public relations firm for 20 years and working with all kinds of businesses, I was used to becoming "an instant expert" on a new subject.

So we acquired all the books, videos, and news articles that would help us make a decision about which treatment I would have. And because I am an inquisitive guy (I was an Associated Press writer at one time) it was easy for me to come up with many questions in a short time.

Now, six years later, having written six books on other topics, I guess it's natural that I should share my information about prostate cancer with others. And I chose to use the style that most appeals to me, questions and answers that are short and understandable.

I realize my limitations—I have had no medical training so I must be careful that I am not dispensing medical recommendations, and that those answers I do provide are accurate.

Two leading New Hampshire urologists, Dr. Gary Dunetz and Dr. Chris Tessier, offered to review this book and without their valuable corrections, advice and suggestions, I would never have written this book.

Two officers of the NH Prostate Cancer Coalition also agreed to review the book. Nancy Kane, our board secretary, is Program Director of the Payson Center for Cancer Care in Concord, NH. Salvatore Magnano, our treasurer, is a prostate cancer survivor and so is his 47 year old son.

Prostate cancer is bad stuff. Urge all your male friends to see their doctor and get screened.

John Sias
September 2007

There's an old saying,
"What you don't know won't hurt you."

Wrong!

What you don't know may just kill you!

TABLE OF CONTENTS

CHAPTER 1
PROSTATE? WHAT'S THAT?

Most of us men don't have the faintest idea where our prostate is and what it does.

And sometimes we have difficulty even pronouncing the word correctly. (It's prostate, not prostrate.)

So what's the prostate?

It's a gland.

What's a gland?

An organ that secretes fluid.

How big is it?

About the size of a walnut.

How big can it grow when it's enlarged?

The size of a lemon.

Where's my prostate located?

Below your bladder and next to your rectum.

It's about three inches from your anus.

What's the function of my prostate?
The biggest job of this little gland is to provide
part of the fluid that makes up your semen.

Where is sperm produced?
In the testicles.

How is my prostate like an apple?
A core runs through the middle of it. This core is actually
more like a tube. This tube is called the *urethra*. All the
urine from your bladder must run through the urethra.

**What two major systems in my body
does my prostate influence?**
Your urinary system. And your reproductive
system. (Two important ones!)

After the reproductive years, what benefit is the prostate?
It prevents infection.

To be fertile, (to make babies) do I need my prostate?
Yes.

Do I need my prostate to be potent? (to get an erection)
No.

The prostate is the source of three common major health problems that affect men. What are they?
Enlargement of the prostate, called BPH.
Prostatitis, a painful inflammation of the prostate.
And prostate cancer.

What's a urologist?
A surgeon who specializes in treating diseases of
the urinary tract and the male reproductive system.
Which, of course, includes the prostate gland.

When should I see a urologist?
Whenever your primary care doctor recommends it.

Have you talked to your doctor about screening?

CHAPTER 2
PROSTATE CANCER CAN KILL YOU

Normal cells divide and grow in an orderly way. This helps to keep the body in good condition. However, sometimes cells divide too rapidly. They grow out of control and form a mass called a tumor.

By the time a tumor has grown to the size of a pea, it has doubled about 30 times. How many cancer cells does the pea-sized tumor contain?
Over 1 billion.

Can a tumor be either benign or malignant?
Yes, either one.

What's a malignant tumor called?
Cancer.

What's dangerous about cancer?
It can invade nearby tissues and organs.

What else can cancer cells do?
They can spread throughout your body.
And then start new tumors.

What's prostate cancer?
It's a malignant tumor found on your prostate gland.

What's so bad about getting prostate cancer?
Well…it could kill you!

**Is PC (prostate cancer) the most common
internal cancer among men?**
Yes. It accounts for 10% of all cancer-related deaths.

How many men each year discover they have PC?
More than 200,000, says the American Cancer Society.

**How many men will be diagnosed with
PC during their lifetime?**
One in 6.

**How many new cases of PC does the American
Cancer Society estimate for 2007?**
218,890.

**How often is a man, somewhere in
the US, diagnosed with PC?**
Every three minutes a new case is detected.

**The number of PC diagnoses has tripled
in the last 15 years. True or false?**
True, mainly because of early detection.

How often does PC appear in a man younger than 46?
Rarely. The typical age for being diagnosed with PC is 69.

**For males of all ages, what is the leading
cause of death by cancer?**
Lung cancer, but PC is second.

What is the leading cause of death by cancer for men over 50?
PC.

How many men die of PC each year?
The forecast for 2007 is 27,400. But that's
DOWN from 43,000 in 1993.

How many male deaths in 2007 will be due to PC?
Every year, one of every 34 men who die will die of PC.

How often does a man somewhere in the US die from PC?
One every 16 minutes.

What's the chance of my dying from PC?
3%. Of every 100 men who die, three will die of PC.

If I get PC, will it affect my job?

Losing your job or losing the opportunity to advance is one of the major concerns of most cancer victims.

What's it like to die of PC?
Often there are liver problems, brain problems, bone fractures and severe bone pain, and comas.

Is it painful?
Doctors' ability to control the effects of PC, pain, nausea etc., has progressed so that most victims do not suffer horribly as was often the situation 10 years ago.

What's a major reason that thousands of us men die each year of PC?
We may have a problem with our prostate but we're afraid to visit our doctor. The cause of the problem could be simple, but because we're afraid, thousands of early cases of PC go undetected, grow, spread throughout the body, and lead to pain and death.

Is it always fatal?
Fortunately, NO. For many men, PC may not worsen as a man grows older. In these cases where the cancer does advance, it's usually curable if caught early enough.

Is it true that fewer men are dying from PC each year?
Yes! And a leading reason is that more men are being screened annually. Doctors are detecting PC earlier.

The vast majority of men diagnosed today with PC, *and then treated*, will live just as long as men who never have the disease. True or false?
True.

What's the 5-year survival rate for PC that is confined to my prostate and has not escaped my prostate?
95%, just about the same as if you had no PC at all.

How many men in the US are PC survivors?
1.8 million.

Since 1992, the US has recorded a 30% decline in age-specific deaths for PC. True or false?
True.

The overall five-year survival rate for PC patients *who have been treated*, is 99%. And the 10-year survival rate is 95%. True or false?
True.

Most men die *with* PC rather than *from* it. True or false?
True.

Doctors are not able to accurately predict which patients will die from PC and which will not. True or false?
False. For many men, doctors are able to predict the outcome.

If you have a life expectancy of fewer than 10 years, is screening likely to benefit you?
No.

Some doctors tell their patients not to worry about PC in that, "Most men have PC some time in their life, but few die from it." What's your reaction?
Sure, most men who have PC do not die from it. But 3% do. Do *you* want to be in that 3%???

Have you talked to your doctor about screening?

CHAPTER 3
WHAT'S MY RISK?

PC is an Equal Opportunity disease. It strikes the rich and the poor, the short and the tall, the smart and the not-so-smart.

How many men have "clinical evidence" of PC?
2.2 million.

What's my chance of developing "clinically evident" PC?
About 1 out of 6.

What are the three major risk factors?
Age, being African-American, and having
a history of PC in your family.

Is PC an "old man's disease"?
Hardly. Even though the older you get, the more at risk you are.

**More than 70% of PCs are diagnosed
in men over 65. True or false?**
True.

For men in their 70s, what's the risk?
A man in his mid- to late-70s is 130 times more likely
to develop PC than a man in his mid- to late- 40s.

So should only older men be concerned with PC?
PC can strike younger men in their 40s and 50s,
especially if there is a family history of PC.

For men 40-59, what's the risk of getting PC?
1 in 44.

What percent of all PC cases are in men over age 50?
95%.

What's my chance of getting PC according to my age?

Birth to 39	1%	1 in 12,000
40-59	2%	1 in 44
60-79	14%	1 in 7
Lifetime	17%	1 in 6

Which race is most at risk for PC?
An African-American man is more likely to get PC, more likely
to get a severe form of PC, more likely to have PC recur after
treatment, and more likely to die from PC than any other race.

**If I'm an African American, what's my chance
of getting PC during my lifetime?**
If you live to be 80, it's 1 out of 4.

Which race of men is most likely to have its PC diagnosed at an advanced age?

African-American.

Are African-American men more likely to die of PC than white American men?

Yes. Almost twice as likely.

How much more likely is a black man with PC likely to die, than a white man?

About 70% more likely. Nobody knows why.

If one family member has PC, how much is my risk increased?

Your risk doubles.

If two family members have PC, how much is my risk increased?

2 to 5 times.

Does it make any difference if PC in my family history is on the side of my mother or my father?

No, your risk is the same.

Which nation has the highest rate of PC in the world?

It's really no contest. American men have the highest rate.

Where in the world is PC most prevalent?
North America, northwestern Europe. Less so in Asia,
Africa, Central America, and South America.

**Deaths from PC are highest in northeast US
and lowest in the southwest. True or false?**
True. Again, nobody knows why.

Which occupations have the highest rate of PC?
Painters, printers, rubber workers, electroplaters,
battery makers, chemical workers, and farmers.

**Who are some celebrities who have been
diagnosed with PC over the last few years?**
Golfer Arnie Palmer. Gen. Norman Schwarzkopf. Baseball
player Stan Musial. Wall Street wizard Mike Milken.
Former Yankees manager Joe Torre. Former Intel CEO
Andy Grove. Actors Sidney Poitier, Charlton Heston,
Jerry Lewis, and Sean Connery. TV personality Ed Ames.
Presidential candidates Senator Bob Dole and Senator
John Kerry and former NY Mayor Rudy Giuliani.

**What do these two have in common? Russian Roulette and
a man's chance of getting PC sometime during his life?**
Both are 1 out of 6.

Have you talked to your doctor about screening?

CHAPTER 4

WHAT ARE THE SYMPTOMS?

Early PC doesn't give off any warning signs.

What are the symptoms of early PC?
When PC is in its early stage (and the cancer is small), there are no symptoms. This is the time when a cure is most possible. And that is exactly why you need to have an annual screening!

PC is usually slow growing. How slow?
Two of every three men with PC never develop any symptoms.

Should I wait until I have symptoms before I get screened?
Absolutely not! Having symptoms might mean you have PC and that it has grown to be incurable.

If a man with PC in its early stages feels perfectly well and has no symptoms, how can his cancer be detected?
The only way to detect tiny amounts of PC is to be screened annually.

Does PC give off ANY warning signals?

Not when it's small. That's why you can't wait around for symptoms. How else will you know if you have PC?

Women are instructed to examine their breasts each month to help detect cancer. Can PC be detected through self-examination?

No.

PC is more often discovered through screening than through symptoms. True or false?

True. Unless you have advanced PC, you are not likely to have any symptoms.

Most men are diagnosed when their PC is NOT causing symptoms. True or false?

True. And the reason is because more PCs are detected early, before they escape from the prostate.

What is advanced PC?

Cancer that probably was detected late and has escaped from the prostate and is now incurable. The cancer can now only be "controlled."

What are the symptoms of advanced PC?

Blood in your urine or your ejaculate.
Many of the same symptoms as BPH (see below).
Severe pain in your back, pelvis, hip or thighs.

Impotence. Or less rigid erections than you used to have.

Less fluid in your ejaculations.

Weight loss.

Decreased appetite.

What causes these symptoms in advanced PC?

Some symptoms can be caused by the urethra (the tube that travels through the middle of the prostate gland, carrying urine from the bladder) being squeezed.

Are there any of these symptoms that will tell me I definitely have PC?

No.

Can every symptom for PC be attributed to some other cause?

Yes. For example, you could have severe pain in your back, pelvis, hips, or thighs. This could be from PC. Or it could be from arthritis, which is much more common than PC that has spread.

What is BPH? (Benign Prostatic Hypertrophy)

Enlargement of the prostate. Our testicles produce testosterone, the key male sex hormone As a man grows older, it's common for his prostate to grow larger. Often this causes urinary problems.

What are the symptoms of BPH?

A decreased rate of flow.

Need to urinate often, maybe several times an hour.

Having to wait for the urinary stream to start.

A sudden need to urinate.

Need to urinate often during the night.

Starting and stopping.

Constant feeling of a full bladder.

Dribbling after you urinate.

If I am a young man and I have urinary symptoms like those above, should I see my doctor?

Yes. These symptoms are often associated with BPH. BPH usually appears after age 60, but may appear earlier.

Does BPH lead to cancer?

No. There is no correlation between PC and BPH.

How common is BPH?

Very. 350,000 of us will develop BPH this year. And 8 of every 10 men will eventually have an enlarged prostate.

What is my risk of getting BPH?

20% of us in our 50s will get BPH.

60% in our 60s.

70% by age 70.

Have you talked to your doctor about screening?

CHAPTER 5
CAN I PREVENT PC?

A healthy life style sure helps.

Does anyone know exactly what causes PC?
No, but some researchers believe that diet plays a role.

Is there any sure way to prevent PC?
No.

How can my diet help fight PC?
Many believe that a good diet helps prevent PC from starting in the first place. And slows the growth of PC that's already begun.

Are there any specific foods that help reduce the risk of getting PC?
You might be able to lower your risk if you eat less red meat and fat, and eat more vegetables, fruits, and grains. Foods high in lycopene are thought to be very helpful. Tomatoes, especially products containing cooked tomatoes, like pizza. Pink grapefruit and watermelon also contain lycopene. A diet that's good for your heart is also good for your prostate.

What else can I do?
Exercise. Reduce stress.

Is obesity a factor in getting PC?
Overweight men run a 30% greater risk than those
within 10% of their ideal body weight.

Might vitamin A supplements increase my risk of getting PC?
It's possible. Check with your doctor.

**I read that men living in Asia hardly ever die of PC, and
women living in Asia hardly ever die of breast cancer. But
when they move to the US, their risk increases. Why?**
They begin to eat fatty foods, put on weight, and exercise
less. They start getting the same diseases we have.

**Some of us may inherit normal genes which have a
tendency to turn cancerous when they are set off by some
"outside factor." What are some of these outside factors?**
High fat diet, lots of red meat, too little
fiber, and environmental pollution.

What role in getting PC does a man's heredity play?
About 15%.

Have you talked to your doctor about screening?

CHAPTER 6
EARLY DETECTION

Discover your cancer early, before it has escaped outside your prostate gland.

Does screening make it more likely that your PC will be found at an early stage? And that it will be curable?
Yes to both questions.

How does PC compare to other cancers I might get?
It usually grows slowly and if you detect it early
and confine it, the chance of cure is great.

How fast does PC grow?
On average, it takes 2-4 years to double in size. This rate
of growth is much slower than breast or colon cancer.

**What advantage is it to me if my doctor
detects PC early rather than late?**
If your cancer grows to a certain size, it can easily escape from
the prostate. It then can spread to nearby seminal vesicles
and lymph nodes. And then into your bloodstream.
When that happens, you've got serious problems.

If the doctor detects my PC early, what are my chances of being cured?
9 out of 10.

What harm can PC do if it's left untreated?
All cancers will grow and spread. Also your cancer could squeeze and obstruct your urethra (the tube that travels through the prostate, carrying urine from the bladder) and this could cause problems.

Do all men have an opportunity to be screened annually?
No. All men in the US do not have equal access to good medical care, especially those who live in the inner city and those in rural areas. A man's financial ability and health insurance are also major factors.

Is it true that nearly all men will develop PC if they live long enough, even though their cancer may never cause symptoms or even be diagnosed?
Yes.

What happens when the cancer cells escape from my prostate?
There are millions of them and they can flee to other parts of your body. Some cells (and you need only one) might get into your bloodstream. Then they could attack your bones, lymph nodes, liver, bladder, rectum, and other organs unless treatment is able to halt the spread.

When PC spreads outside the prostate, is it curable?
Not usually.

How much time will cancers need before they spread?
This will vary from man to man. Genetic
factors play a major role.

**Why are so many PCs diagnosed incurable
when they are first detected?**
One answer is that the cancer was detected too late. If the
man had annual screenings, the PC would probably have been
detected earlier when it had a high chance of being curable.

If cancer cells escape from my prostate, are operations feasible?
When cells spread, they spread to many different places in
your body. Removing all these cancerous cells in all these
new locations is impossible. However, some cells which
do escape may not be able to live outside the prostate.

**How many of us men are walking around
today with PC which is about to spread or is
already spreading throughout our body?**
About 1 million.

**How would I know that my PC is so far
advanced that it's not curable?**
Your doctor would perform an evaluation which would
include PSA, bone scan, x-rays and a physical exam.

If my cancer is in its late stages when doctors first detect it (it's incurable then), can doctors usually control it, even if they can't cure it?

Yes, for a limited time.

Why do most men know so little, or nothing, about PC until they get it?

First, the public, especially men, simply are not very aware of PC. Secondly, we humans, especially men, too often neglect our health. Third, we just don't take advantage of preventative measures.

So, if I want to increase my odds of surviving PC, what should I do?

Current guidelines recommend that all men have an annual PSA test starting at age 50, provided they do not have any major medical problems and can expect to live at least 10 years. And get screened every year. That way you can detect cancer when it's early, and treat it before it escapes from your prostate.

Have you talked to your doctor about screening?

CHAPTER 7
SCREENING

Give yourself a birthday present.

What is screening?
Using two tests to see if you have PC. The digital rectal exam (DRE) and the PSA (Prostate Specific Antigen) blood test.

Is screening for men who have symptoms of PC?
No. Screening is for men who have NO symptoms. If you have symptoms, that means you should have started screening years ago.

Any other reasons to get screened?
Another good reason you should have an annual screening is that it provides your doctor with a base line (a marker). If he has a base line, he can compare your condition from year to year. A steady and continuously rising PSA is a strong indicator of trouble.

Who needs to be screened?
All men who don't want PC, and who have a life expectancy of at least 10 years.

When should I begin screening?

When you reach 50, you need to be screened every year. However if you are African-American or have a family history of PC, you should begin screening at age 40-45. Most cancers are slow growing. But some are fast growing and once they get up a head of steam, they spread like wildfire.

Is there one specific test that will tell me, for sure, if I have PC?

No. The DRE and the PSA tests are not foolproof, but they are the best indicators we have.

Why do I need both a PSA test and a digital rectal exam (DRE)?

Because one test detects cancers that the other test sometimes fails to detect.

Should I have my PSA test and digital rectal exam (DRE) at the same time?

Sure, but ask the doctor to do the DRE after he draws blood for the PSA test. Sometimes the DRE activity temporarily elevates the PSA and gives you an erroneous high reading.

If my doctor screens only by the digital rectal method, what percent of PC cases will he detect?

Only 20%.

Why such a low number?
Mainly because most small cancers are too
small to be felt by your doctor.

**When my doctor screens with both DRE and
PSA, what percent of cancers will he
detect?**
About 60%.

**Is the PSA test a routine part of a standard
battery of blood tests that I might have?**
Not necessarily. For example, if you have a
typical "annual physical" the PSA test might not
be included. To be sure, ask for the test.

Who will usually perform my screening?
Your primary care doctor.

I'm not sure I've been screened. How do I find out?
Just call your doctor and ask him.

**Before I get screened, do I have to take any pills or laxative?
Do I have to undergo any preparations of any kind?**
No.

**Will I have any after-affects from the PSA
or DRE tests? Any pain? Nausea?**
None from the PSA, but mild discomfort from the DRE test.

How many men reach their 50th birthday each year, and should begin screening?
1.7 million.

What percent of men of screening age have a PSA blood test and the DRE on an annual basis?
Only 50%, says the National Prostate Cancer Coalition.

If I am not expected to live more than 10 years, because of other health issues, should I bother with screening?
Probably not. In that time, the normal cancer won't grow large enough to be a problem. Chances are that you'll die of something other than PC.

Who is in favor of doctors offering screenings to men at age 50 who are at average risk?
Advocates include authorities like the American Cancer Society, American Urological Association, and the US Food and Drug Administration.

How can I remember to have an annual screening?
Try using some annual event like your birthday or anniversary.

Have you talked to your doctor about screening?

CHAPTER 8
FEELING FOR BUMPS WITH DRE

It's not fun, but it's no big deal.

What is a digital rectal exam? (DRE)
It's an examination (the E). It's an exam via your rectum (the R). And it's done by your doctor using his gloved digit (finger) (the D) to feel if you have any abnormality on your prostate gland.

What's the purpose of the DRE? What's the doctor trying to do?
The doctor is feeling if there are any bumps or areas of increased firmness on your prostate. Bumps on your prostate strongly indicate cancer.

What are these bumps like?
Hold up your left hand. With the index finger of your right hand, feel the fleshy skin at the base of your left thumb. This is what a normal prostate feels like. Now, with that same index finger, feel the knuckle of your left thumb. This is how a cancer feels, a hard lump. Your doctor is feeling to see if there are any of these hard lumps on your prostate.

How big are these bumps?

The size of a pea. Or larger.

Other than a bump, what might the doctor be watching for?

He could be looking for subtle changes of increased firmness of your prostate. Or changes in the symmetry or shape of your prostate. Or if your prostate is extending beyond its normal location.

How conclusive is the DRE?

It's not perfect because it's based on the skill and judgment of the physician. Some physicians simply are more skillful and better judges than others.

Can the doctor distinguish early stage cancers (when the potential for cure is the greatest?)

No.

Is the doctor able to feel all around the prostate?

No. He can only feel the outer side of your prostate gland.

On which side of your prostate is a tumor most likely to occur?

Fortunately, on the outer side, which is the only side your doctor can feel in the DRE. The other side, the inner side, is up against your bladder. Your doctor is unable to feel that side because he has no access to that side.

What is a limitation of the DRE?
It detects only cancers which are large
enough to be felt by the doctor.

**What percent of cancers are located in areas of the prostate
that the doctor is physically unable to reach with his finger?**
30% to 40% of cancers go undetected because
they're out of the reach of the doctor. Or they
are so small he is unable to feel them.

**If I have a positive DRE, what is my
chance that I actually have PC?**
Maybe as high as 50%. But it depends
on just what the DRE reveals.

If my DRE is positive, what should I do?
Have your PSA tested. And talk to your doctor
about the possible need for a biopsy.

**What if it's negative? Does a normal
DRE mean you do *not* have PC?**
No.

If I have the DRE, why do I need the PSA test too?
The PSA test is more sensitive and more specific
than the DRE and can find more cancers.

So if I have a PSA test, then I don't need the DRE, too, right?

Wrong. Sometimes the DRE can find cancers
in men with normal PSA levels.
25% of men with PC have a low PSA. The PSA is not foolproof.

When the doctor screens with both the DRE and the PSA, what is the detection rate?

60%.

Does the DRE hurt?

No. But, but it's uncomfortable.

You say it doesn't hurt. But when my doctor gives me a DRE, it always hurts. What should I do?

You could try a different doctor. Some doctors
are just better than others at giving a DRE.

What can I do to make my DRE painless?

Bend over the edge of the examining table. It's
a better position than lying on your side.

Is it necessary? I really don't like it!

Yes. You don't like the DRE? Join the rest of all the
men in the world who ever had a DRE! Guess what?
Women don't like mammograms either. Or Pap tests.

Have you talked to your doctor about screening?

CHAPTER 9
PSA, THE GREAT INDICATOR

It's not perfect, but it's still the best we have.

What is PSA?

It's a protein. It's made by the prostate in large amounts. Although it's made in the prostate, it leaks into the blood stream and doctors can detect it and measure it in a simple blood test. The important point is that high levels of PSA can *indicate* the presence of cancer.

What do the letters PSA stand for?

Prostate-specific antigen.

Is PSA produced only by the prostate gland?

Yes.

The larger a man's prostate gland, the more PSA is produced. True or false?

True.

What does PSA do?

It liquefies sperm so it can travel up the female reproductive tract.

What is a PSA test?

It's simply a blood test.

Where does the blood come from in a PSA test?

Most often when you have a routine physical exam, your doctor sends your blood sample to a lab and asks the lab to perform a series of tests. Often the PSA is included in the list of tests to be done. Ask your doctor to be sure it is.

How long will it take to get the results of my PSA test?

Two days to a week.

How much does a PSA test cost?

About $55. This is often covered by health insurance companies. Also, some hospitals offer free screenings once a year.

What exactly does the PSA test accomplish for me?

The PSA test is an *indicator* that you might have PC. It's only an indicator. It's not foolproof. But at present, it's the *best* indicator we have.

***Before* PSA testing was used, what percent of those cancers which were detected, had already spread beyond the victim's prostate and were incurable?**

70%.

After **PSA testing was used extensively, what percent of cancers were detected, and proved curable?**

70%, just the opposite.

Why is PSA such a good indicator of PC?

Under normal conditions, PSA is disposed of through ducts in our prostate. However, in a man with PC, the PSA gets into the blood stream more readily, and leaks out of the prostate. Then doctors can measure PSA in the blood stream.

Without PSA screening, about 40% of PCs are not detected until they have spread too far to be curable. True or false?

True.

What's a normal PSA?

0-4 nanograms per milliliter. (ng/ml)

What does your PSA level tell your doctor?

PSA 4-10	slightly elevated, may indicate early cancer confined to prostate
11-20	moderately elevated, cancer may have spread locally
over 20	highly elevated, probable widespread cancer invading lymph nodes and other tissues

Do PSA results alone provide sufficient information either to: Diagnose PC? Rule out PC?

No, but a high PSA is an *indicator* of PC.

If my PSA is 0-4, is this a guarantee that I do not have PC?
No.

What's my chance of having PC with a 4-10 reading?
25%.

**What percent of men over 50 who are
screened will have an elevated PSA?**
Only 10% to 15%.

Of those 10%, how many will have PC?
About one-third will have prostate cancer.

What can cause a high PSA reading besides PC?
Infection, inflammation, enlarged prostate (BPH),
a drug you're taking, ejaculation within the last 48
hours, a biopsy, a mistake in the medical lab.

What is a "baseline" PSA?
It's the first PSA screening you have. All subsequent PSA
tests can be measured against this "baseline" to determine
if your PSA is rising. And how fast it is rising.

Why is it important to know how fast your PSA is rising?
Velocity, the rate at which your PSA is
rising, is a strong indicator of PC.

Doctors believe that the overall PSA level may be less important than the rate at which the PSA level rises. True or false?

True.

Do all PCs grow at the same rate?

No. Most are slow growing. But some are fast-growing, aggressive, and deadly.

When a doctor first detects PC, can he tell whether the PC is slow growing or fast growing?

No.

For men with a high initial PSA of 10 or more, is velocity a consideration?

No.

When was PSA discovered?

In the mid-1970s by Japanese scientists.

When did PSA testing begin?

In the early 1980s.

Today, men are diagnosed earlier than previously. How much earlier?

Five years earlier, according to the National Cancer Institute.

When did the American Cancer Society recommend that doctors use the PSA test as part of a routine screening? 1992.

In early May of 2007, the New York Times said that American Urological Association will soon release revised guidelines. What will these guidelines hope to do?

- Reduce the cost of screening.
- Reduce unnecessary biopsies.
- Reduce unnecessary prostate surgeries.
- Reduce the cost per life saved.
- Reduce overall deaths from PC.

What will these AUA guidelines suggest?

- That doctors no longer rely on a single PSA reading.
- That doctors focus on changes in PSA levels over time.
- Lower the PSA level for requesting a biopsy.
- That men get a baseline PSA test at age 40.
- That men get a PSA test at 40 and 45.
- That men get an annual PSA test at age 50 until 70.

Have you talked to your doctor about screening?

CHAPTER 10
PSA SAVES LIVES

Are you willing to gamble with <u>your</u> life?

You'll probably hear some people argue that the PSA screening is not effective. Here's what they might say.

- Some very early stage cancers found by screening might never cause you a problem.

- Many men do have PC but their cancer does not escape the prostate.

- Regular PSA testing could spot the "incidental" cancers that are present in 30% of men over 50. These incidental cancers do not need treatment.

- Some physicians are not sure how to interpret PSA readings.

- If the PSA is high, the chance that you have PC is relatively small.

- Inconclusive or false test results could cause confusion and anxiety.

- Normal test results can give a false sense of security when, in fact, cancer is really present.

- Widespread PSA testing could encourage thousands of men to have unnecessary and expensive biopsies. And these biopsies might lead to unnecessary treatments.

- You may become so focused on "Get rid of that cancer" that you decide to have treatments, even if the risks outweigh the probable benefits.

- Treatments can have undesirable side effects, such as urinary and sexual problems.

- Tests, such as a biopsy, can cause bleeding and infection.

- Two of every three men who have an abnormal PSA will undergo further tests which are invasive and sometimes frightening. Yet these further tests will show the man is perfectly healthy.

- These further tests can be expensive.

- Some cancers are so small they fail to raise the PSA or fail to be felt during the DRE.

- Screening does not necessarily translate into longer lives.

- The National Cancer Institute, the country's leading cancer research organization, takes no position on regular screening. They say there is no clear-cut balance between the number of lives saved by early detection and the number of lives affected by unnecessary treatment.

But here's the other side of the argument.

- PC is silent. It gives no warning in its early stage. There are no symptoms until the PC grows outside the prostate. It is then incurable. PSA screening increases the chance of finding PC **before** it escapes the prostate and spreads throughout your body.

- You need both the DRE and the PSA because the DRE alone is not foolproof. The doctor can feel only half your prostate. And he cannot feel an early cancer. The PSA can also detect different cancers than the DRE.

- In America, fewer men are dying from PC each year. This is largely because the PSA test is helping doctors diagnose and treat PC earlier, at a more curable stage. In 1995 (before PSA testing was popular), **40,000 men died** of PC. In 2006 (after several years of PSA testing), the number of deaths was **down to 27,000**.

- A PSA test will detect PC about **5-10 years earlier** than a DRE alone.

- Before PSA testing was widely used, and the DRE was the only method of detecting PC, almost **75% of those cancers detected were advanced** (neither readily treatable nor curable).

- Now that PSA tests are commonplace, almost **75% are detected in the early stage**.

- Regularly scheduled PSA testing virtually *eliminates* the diagnosis of advanced PC.

- Back in 1988-91, before PSA was widely used, a man had a *12% chance of dying* from PC within five years, according to studies at Walter Reed Army Hospital. After PSA was widely used (1995-98), another study was ordered and found the death rate had dropped to *1%.*

- Earlier diagnosis translates into higher rates of cure.

- 30-50% of cancers detected by PSA screening would never have been apparent otherwise, says Johns Hopkins Medical Center.

So, look at it this way. Sure, some of the negative arguments sound good, but, if you have not had both the DRE and the PSA, *How can you be <u>sure</u> you don't have Prostate Cancer right now?* If you are over 50 and want to live another 10-30 years, *get screened now*.

Have you talked to your doctor about screening?

CHAPTER 11
BIOPSY, PROOF POSITIVE

**What is the best way to find out whether
a high PSA level indicates PC?**
Though not perfect, a biopsy is the best way.

What's a biopsy?
The doctor takes tiny samples from your prostate. He sends
them to the lab where other doctors, called pathologists,
examine these samples to see if they are cancerous.

What's important about a biopsy?
It's the *only* way you'll *really* know if you have PC. The
DRE and PSA might ***indicate*** you have PC. But until you
have a biopsy and cancer is found, you will not be sure.

**Current guidelines recommend that a man have a
biopsy if his PSA level exceeds 4, or if the PSA has risen
significantly between the last two PSA tests. True or false?**
True.

Is a biopsy a fun thing to do?

Hell, no. But neither is a broken bone, or a cut requiring several stitches. And the biopsy, including the ultrasound, is all over in 15 minutes.

Does it hurt?

Hurt, no. Uncomfortable, yes.

Where does the doctor perform the biopsy?

In his office. See, it's not such a big deal.

How long does a biopsy take?

About 12 minutes.

What does ultrasound do?

The doctor uses it to estimate the size of tumors on your prostate. He also uses it to guide the needle during a biopsy. The ultrasound exam takes about five minutes.

How many "samples" should my urologist take from my prostate?

At least 10. Typical number is 12.

What are the dimensions of the 12 samples taken in a typical biopsy?

Each is about ½ inch long and 1/6 inches wide.

What does a biopsy (pathology) report tell?

      1. the type of cancer

      2. the grade of the cancer

      3. the volume of the cancer

Is it possible for a biopsy to miss my cancer?

Yes. Sometimes the biopsy will miss the cancer even when it's there because such a small amount of tissue is taken in the samples.

What's the chance that my biopsy will be positive (that I have PC)?

A recent trial showed that of men with a PSA of less than 4, who were biopsied, 15% of them had PC. If you have a PSA between 4 and 10, there's a 25% chance that your biopsy will prove that you have PC.

After studying the results of my biopsy, my doctor tells me I have PC. Should I get a second opinion?

Many men seek a second opinion.

If my biopsy is positive, how soon do I have to act?

If your cancer is a normal one, it's probably been growing for 10 years. You do not need to make any panic decisions, but neither can you procrastinate.

If my biopsy is negative, is that a guarantee that I do not have PC?

No, unfortunately. If your doctor felt a hard lump during his DRE exam, a "negative biopsy" might mean that the biopsy exam missed the cancer. Consult your doctor about a second biopsy.

How many biopsies are performed in the US each year?

About 800,000.

Have you talked to your doctor about screening?

CHAPTER 12
DIAGNOSING. DISCOVERING THAT YOU HAVE PC

More than 4 out of every 10 men diagnosed with prostate cancer will have cancer that has spread beyond the prostate gland.

How often is a new case of PC diagnosed?
Every 3 minutes some man gets the bad news that he has PC. Hopefully, the doctor detected it early.

What's the average age that men are diagnosed with PC?
69.

When are cancer cells detectable?
Sometimes not until there are several million of them.

What does "curable" mean?
Your cancer has been detected in its early stage, when it's still treatable. But "cured" is not a word that doctors often use when referring to PC. Why? Because it is not possible to be 100% sure that the PC will not return.

What percent of all prostate cancers are discovered in the local and regional stages?
91%.

What is "local"?
When PC is still confined to your prostate gland.

What is "regional"?
When PC has spread to nearby areas, but not to distant sites such as your bones.

When PC spreads outside the prostate gland, where does it usually spread first?
To the pelvic lymph nodes.

What is the purpose of the lymphatic system?
It defends the body against disease and infection.

If PC spreads to the bones, is it still called prostate cancer?
Yes. Even when a cancer has spread to a new place in your body, it is still called by the same (original) name. For example, when a woman has breast cancer and it spreads to her lungs, it's still called breast cancer.

If I'm treated when my cancer is diagnosed early, what are my chances of living at least five more years?
87%.

If my cancer has already spread to distant parts of my body at the time of my diagnosis, what are my chances of survival?
The 5-year survival rate then is 34%.

Do all PCs grow at the same rate?
No. Most are slow-growing. Some can take 10-12 years before they are large enough to be detected. Then another six years before they double in size.

What percent of cancers diagnosed are considered slow growing?
20-54%.

Is there any guarantee that even a slow growing cancer won't eventually be life-threatening?
No.

What does "incurable" mean?
Your cancer has escaped your prostate and spread to other parts of your body. These new cancers cannot be killed. Doctors will try to limit your pain.

What percent of PCs are not diagnosed until they have escaped the prostate?
40%.

What is PSA "velocity"?
How fast your PSA is rising between PSA tests.

Do doctors consider PSA velocity to be a better indicator of PC than a single PSA test?
Yes.

Over what period of time is velocity measured? And how many tests?
1 ½ to 2 years, and 2 to 3 PSA tests. However, if a man's PSA is rising, more frequent PSA tests will be ordered.

What about the fast-growing aggressive cancers?
Some men with these cancers will die despite all therapy.

What percent of cancers are considered aggressive upon the first screening?
20%.

How do doctors tell the difference between a typical slow-growing PC and an aggressive, fast-growing PC, the type that's responsible for most of the 27,000 deaths each year?
From the results of your biopsy, doctors rate on the "Gleason" scale how aggressive your cancer is. A Gleason grade of 8, 9 or 10 is aggressive.

What is cancer "grade?"
A measure of how aggressive the cancer is. The lower your Gleason score, the better.

What is cancer "stage"?

The extent of the spread of the cancer. Has
the cancer escaped the prostate and spread to
nearby tissues or other parts of the body?

**The PSA test can help spot PC. But can this
test tell how dangerous the cancer is?**

No. However, the PSA has some ability to correlate with staging.

**Why is it a good idea to get a second opinion
for a man diagnosed with PC?**

Screening and other tests can result in a misdiagnosis
of PC. Accurately diagnosing PC can be tricky.

What is a "second opinion"?

Having another pathologist re-read the slides of your biopsy.

What is a "prognosis?"

It's a prediction of the probable course of your disease.
It tells you how likely you are to recover from PC.

What are the key factors in a prognosis?

1. how large your tumor is
2. the location and extent of your primary tumor
3. your PSA before treatment
4. your Gleason score (how aggressive your
   cancer would likely be if it's not treated).

What's a "favorable prognosis"?

Your PC is likely to respond well to treatment.

What is an "unfavorable prognosis"?

Your PC will probably be difficult to treat and control.

Have you talked to your doctor about screening?

CHAPTER 13
TREATMENT

There are a number of treatment options for prostate cancer, but there is no <u>cure</u> for PC.

How soon after I'm diagnosed for PC, must I make a decision as to which treatment I will select?
PC is generally a slow-growing cancer. Most men take several weeks or months to make their decision.

Do most men feel this decision to be one of the most difficult, confusing, and frustrating decisions they ever made in their entire life?
Absolutely.

How do I decide which treatment is best for me?
- Read every pamphlet and book you can.
- Search the internet.
- Talk with survivors, urologists, radiation oncologists, physicians, friends.
- Attend a support group meeting.
- Search the web sites of the many national organizations specializing in PC.

- Watch videos on PC.
- Read the cancer treatment guidelines.

What information do cancer treatment guidelines offer?
- A list of FAQ (Frequently Asked Questions) that you should consider asking before making a decision.
- A chart listing all treatment choices, the pros and cons of each, side effects of each, and other valuable information.

Where can I obtain these cancer treatment guidelines?
Several national organizations publish a guide. Among them are:
- American Urological Association. Auanet.org
- National Cancer Institute. Cancer.gov
- National Comprehensive Cancer Network. Nccn.org

What questions should I ask?
You can find a list of questions in many of these guidelines. Another complete list is in the American Cancer Society's "Complete Guide to Prostate Cancer" published in 2005 and available free.

I want to talk to other men who have already faced this same situation and who have made a treatment decision. Where can I locate such men who would be willing to talk with me?
Visit a prostate cancer support group in your area. For a list of PC support groups, contact your local hospital. Or American Cancer Society at 1-800-ACS-2345. Or USTOO at 1-800-808 7866. Or look on the web site of your state's Prostate Cancer Coalition.

What are my options for treatment if my cancer has not spread to my lymph nodes and/or bones?
- Watchful waiting
- External beam radiation
- Internal radiation (Seeds, brachytherapy)
- Surgery
- Laparoscopic (robotic) surgery
- Cryotherapy (freezing the DNA)

"Watchful waiting." What is it?
You receive no active treatments such as surgery or radiation. Your doctors closely observe your situation. You probably will have a PSA test and DRE every six months and maybe a biopsy every other year. If you start to have symptoms or if your cancer begins to grow more quickly, you can think about active treatments.

Who is a candidate for watchful waiting?
Older men, and men with less than a 10 year probable life expectancy. Watchful waiting is not a usual choice if you are young, healthy, or have a fast-growing cancer.

Is it natural for surgical specialists, such as urologists, to recommend surgery? And for radiation oncologists to recommend radiation?
Yes, because that is their field of specialty. But a good doctor should present all options.

**Is there one specific treatment that will
guarantee my cancer will never return?**
No.

**Most doctors now feel there are treatments which are best
used for the earliest stage PC. What are these treatments?**
External radiation, radical prostatectomy (surgical removal
of the prostate gland), and radioactive seed implants.

What is the definition of "survival rate"?
The percent of patients who do not die from PC
within 5 years after their cancer is first treated.

**What is the 5-year survival rate for men treated
with surgery, whose PC was still within their
prostate gland when it was discovered?**
Nearly 100%.

**What is the 5-year survival rate for men whose cancers, when
found, had already spread to distant parts of their body?**
Only 34%.

What are my options if I have advanced cancer?
Hormonal therapy and chemotherapy.

Is there any 'best" treatment for every man?
No.

Do all treatments have side effects?

Almost all.

Why do treatments have side effects?

Any drug or treatment that's powerful enough to
kill cancer cells in your body may also be strong
enough to affect your body in other ways.

What are the potential side effects of each treatment?

See the guidelines and the American Cancer
Society book mentioned above.

What types of doctors should I consider consulting?

- Urologist
- Family physician
- Radiation oncologist
- Medical oncologist

Will I offend anyone by consulting other physicians?

No, doctors understand the complexity
and the pressure you are under.

**I've been told if I take hormones (to reduce the size
of my prostate) that I will have "hot flashes" just like
my wife experienced in menopause. Is this true?**

Sure is. And don't expect much sympathy from the opposite sex!

What does treatment cost (over a 6 year period)?

- Androgen deprivation therapy $69,244
- External beam radiation $59,455
- Seeds $35,143

Source: CANCER Jan. 1, 2007

What is a "clinical trial"?

It's a study of a promising new treatment
that might be of value to the patient.

What are my risks in a clinical trial?

No one knows in advance if the treatment will
work. Or what side effects might occur.

Am I free to leave a clinical trial at any time for any reason?

Yes.

Will taking part in a clinical trial prevent me from getting other medical care for my needs?

No. But you have to qualify for a clinical trial because previous conventional treatments have not worked. And the principle treatment of your medical condition may result in an exclusion.

Whose decision is this to be in a clinical trial?

Yours. It's your body, your life.

Is it possible for PC to recur many years after my initial treatment?

Yes, so keep your regular doctor visits. And report any new symptoms such as bone pain or problems with urination.

When will I know that I've made the best decision (for me)?

It will probably be many, many years.

Have you talked to your doctor about screening?

CHAPTER 14
WE MEN

Ignore it. It will go away. Right? Wrong!

Why do we men not talk about our ailments?
A lot of us men think we have to be indestructible.
That's the way we were brought up! When we got
hurt, we were taught to "tough it out." We don't
want to admit our fear or our vulnerability.

Why don't more men get screened annually?
Some of us are "too busy." Others would make any
excuse to avoid seeing a doctor. And some of us
aren't even aware that we ought to get screened.

Why are men so reticent about discussing PC?
It has to do with our sexual potency, our manliness. Besides,
most of us work on the principle of, "I'll learn about it,
if and when if affects me. And not until that time."

**I'm avoiding screening because I'm afraid I'll
learn that I have PC. What should I do?**
A vast majority of those screened do *not* have PC. However,
PC doesn't stop growing just because you aren't ready to deal
with the subject. What you don't know really CAN hurt you.

**In a Louis Harris survey of 4,350 men and women,
what percent of the men said they would wait several
days after "severe chest pains" before seeing a doctor?**
One third of the men said they'd wait. Another
third said they'd never seek help at all.

What percent of the men surveyed had no regular doctor?
One third.

How many American men visited a doctor in the last year?
Fewer than 25%.

**How many of these men had a PC
screening in the previous year?**
Only 4 of every 10, of those over age 50.

**How many had NOT been screened
for PC in the last five years?**
One third.

What percent of Americans think they have little or no control over reducing their risk for cancer?

47%, said the American Cancer Society in January, 2007.

PC is the second leading cause of male cancer deaths. PC can be a long term way to die. Is getting an annual screening (PSA and DRE) worth your time? And if your PSA is high, you might need a biopsy. Is all this worth it?

The DRE takes 20 seconds. The PSA takes 60 seconds. A biopsy, including the ultrasound exam, takes 15 minutes. Compare those 16 minutes to years of possible excruciating pain followed by an early death. The choice is yours!

For those of us who get embarrassed or are actually afraid of a doctor inserting a gloved finger up our rectum, what should we do? Would you rather die?

Some men would. But put things in perspective. Before life is over, you'll own 20 cars, five houses, and six computers. But only one body that's got to last you all your life. Most of us take better care of cars, houses, and computers than our one body.

Which do we men do most often: check the oil, rotate the tires, or get screened?

Check the oil. Winner by a long shot!

What may be the last all-male club in the US?

Those of us who have PC. This is one club women will never be able to join.

Why is PC the male equivalent of breast cancer?

Breast cancer and PC have remarkably similar statistics. The lifetime risk for breast cancer is 1 in 8, for PC 1 in 6. Average age when the cancer is diagnosed is 69 for men, 63 for women. New cases diagnosed annually are 220,000 for PC, and 192,200 for breast cancer.

How do the survival rates and death tolls compare?

Survival rates are somewhat similar. Deaths from breast cancer annually are 44,000 and for PC, they are 27,000.

Why do I hear so much more about breast cancer than PC?

Women are much more comfortable discussing and asking questions about their bodies than we men.

It's a rough day for this mythical couple both age 50. She's just found out that her mammogram is positive and he's found out his PSA is over 4, the top level for normal. Which one is more likely to have cancer?

The husband. His probability is 25%. Hers is 9%.

Have you talked to your doctor about screening?

CHAPTER 15
TAKE CHARGE. A CASE FOR ANNUAL SCREENING

Prostate cancer is the **leading cancer killer** of men over 50: 27,000 deaths in 2006.

Your chance of getting PC sometime during your life is 1 in 6. These are the same odds as **Russian Roulette**.

A high PSA indicates you probably have **some** kind of disease in your prostate.

Annual screening means that cancers can be **detected early**.

Early detection of PC results in the **greatest chance of cure.**

Annual screening will give you peace of mind. It will **reduce your worrying**, "Could _I_ have prostate cancer?"

Annual screenings can provide you a greater degree of **confidence** that if you ever do get PC, it will be detected at the earliest possible time.

Annual screenings can **reduce the worry** of family and friends who are concerned that you might develop PC and that it will be detected too late.

Early detection and early treatment can make a huge difference in the **quality of life** during your retirement years.

Early detection can give you years of **pain free living.**

Not being screened can be a **life or death** difference.

Annual screenings might **save your life.**

A man should do **everything possible** to protect his long-term health. PC seldom causes any symptoms before it becomes **incurable**.

The only practical strategy for avoiding death and suffering is to find the PC and treat it early.

A better screening test than PSA and DRE may be **several years** in the future. In that time, several hundred thousand men will die of PC.

Men who regularly have an annual screening will be among the **first to benefit** when the medical world develops improved screening methods.

Talking to your doctor about screening is **endorsed** by American Cancer Society, American Urological Assn., and American College of Radiology. These are the medical groups which have the most experience in dealing with PC patients.

Have you talked to your doctor about screening?

PROSTATE CANCER INDEX

Number of American men between 50 and 80   27,000,000

Number who will be diagnosed with PC this year   200,000

Number who will die this year   27,000

Risk of men 40-59 getting PC   1 in 53

Risk of men 60-79 getting PC   1 in 7

How often a man dies of PC   every 16 minutes

The number of tests that can
    definitely tell a man if he has PC   0

Detection rate of digital rectal exam   20%

Detection rate of PSA   40%

Detection rate of both together   60%

A man's chance of dying from PC   3%

Age when men should begin annual screening for PC   50

Number of men who will turn 50 this year   1,781,000

Chance of surviving 5 years if
    the cancer escapes from the prostate   40%

Chance of surviving 5 years when
the cancer reaches bone   20%

Caucasian man's chance of being diagnosed with PC   1 in 8

African-American's chance of
being diagnosed with PC   1 in 6

Number of years a detectable
cancer has been growing inside   10

Age at which PC most often is detected   69

SOME SOURCES OF INFORMATION
ABOUT PROSTATE CANCER

BOOKS

100 Questions and Answers about Prostate Cancer,
    Pamela Ellsworth MD, 2003

ABCs of Prostate Cancer, Joseph Oesterling, MD, 1997

Cancer at Your Fingertips, Val Speechley and
    Maxine Rosenfeld, 2001

Complete Guide to Prostate Cancer, American
    Cancer Society, 2005

Coping With Prostate Cancer, Robert Philips, 1994

Guide to Surviving Prostate Cancer, Patrick Walsh MD, 2001

Hit Below the Belt, Ralph Berberich MD, 2001

I Flunked My PSA Test! Ernie Bodai MD, 2002

Living with Cancer, Jeffrey Tobias et al, 2001

Living With Prostate Cancer, David Wynn, 2003

Man to Man, Michael Korda, 1996

My Prostate and Me, William Martin, 1995

Prostate and Cancer, Sheldon Marks MD, 1999

Prostate Cancer for Dummies, Paul Lange MD
    and Christine Adamec, 2003

Prostate Cancer, A Doctor's Personal Triumph, Saralee
    Fine and Robert Fine MD, 1999

Prostate Cancer, A Non-Surgical Perspective,
    Kent Wallner, MD, 1996

Prostate Cancer, A Survivor's Guide, Don Kaltenbach, 1995

Prostate Cancer, Allen E. Salowe, 1997

Prostate Cancer: A Comprehensive Guide for
    Patients, R. Persad etc, 2002

Prostate Cancer: A Family Guide, 2003

Prostate Disease, W. Scott McDougal MD 1996

Prostrate Cancer Answer Book, Marion Morra, 1996

Surviving Prostate Cancer, E. Fuller Torrey, Yale U. Press, 2006

The Prostate, Yosh Taguchi MD, 2001

The Prostate: A Guide for Men and the Women Who
    Love Them, Patrick Walsh, MD,1997

The Prostate Book: An Owner's Manual, Dr. Peter Scadino, 2005

Understanding Male Sexual Health, Hyppocratic, 1993

What Can I Do? My Husband Has Prostate Cancer, Bev Farmer, 1995

PAMPHLETS AND BROCHURES

After Diagnosis: Prostate Cancer, ACS, 2002

Cancer Survivors Network, ACS, 2003

Facts on Prostate Cancer, ACS, 2002

Guidelines for the Early Detection of Cancer, ACS, 2003

Know Your Options, US TOO, 2000

Man to Man support groups, ACS, 2003

Managing Incontinence, ACS, 2001

Prostate Cancer, Treatment Guidelines, ACS, 2000

Should I Be Tested for Prostate Cancer? ACS, 2003

Treatment Choices for Men Living With Advanced Prostate Cancer, Cancer Care, 2004

Where to Turn, ACS, 2002

www.ingramcontent.com/pod-product-compliance
Lightning Source LLC
Chambersburg PA
CBHW021230280526
45784CB00005B/2045